The Ketogenic Lectin Free Cookbook

Easy and Wholesome Keto Lectin Free Recipes to
Lose Weight Quickly and Heal Your Body
(Lose Up to 20 Pounds in 28 Days)

By [Alisia Walker]

© **Copyright 2018 by Alisia Walker- All rights reserved.**

This document is geared towards providing exact and reliable information in regards to the topic and issue covered. The publication is sold with the idea that the publisher is not required to render accounting, officially permitted, or otherwise, qualified services. If advice is necessary, legal or professional, a practiced individual in the profession should be ordered.

From a Declaration of Principles which was accepted and approved equally by a Committee of the American Bar Association and a Committee of Publishers and Associations.

In no way is it legal to reproduce, duplicate, or transmit any part of this document in either electronic means or in printed format. Recording of this publication is strictly prohibited and any storage of this document is not allowed unless with written permission from the publisher. All rights reserved.

The information provided herein is stated to be truthful and consistent, in that any liability, in terms of inattention or otherwise, by any usage or abuse of any policies, processes, or directions contained within is the solitary and utter responsibility of the recipient reader. Under no circumstances will any legal responsibility or blame be held against the publisher for any reparation, damages, or monetary loss due to the information herein, either directly or indirectly.

Respective authors own all copyrights not held by the publisher.

Introduction 1

Understanding the Keto Lectin-Free Diet 2

    What Is the Keto Lectin-Free Diet 2

    Keto Lectin-Free Diet Guidelines 3

    Food That You Can Consume 3

    Food to Avoid 5

    The Benefits of The Keto Lectin-Free Diet 7

Breakfast Recipes 9

    Avocado Smoothie 9

    Breakfast Burger with Avocado 10

    Cauliflower and Ground Beef Skillet 11

    Avocado Salmon Breakfast Cups 12

    Cauliflower Fritters 13

    Coconut Flour Porridge 14

    Avocado Smoothie with Coconut Milk, Ginger, And Turmeric 15

    Shrimp Omelet 16

    Steak and Eggs 17

    Guacamole Eggs 18

    Bacon and Basil Egg Omelet 19

    Keto Strawberry Breakfast Smoothie 20

    Breakfast Sausage Casserole 21

    Coconut Cherry Vanilla Smoothie 22

    Bacon Spinach Frittata 23

Lunch Recipes 24

    Lemon Balsamic Chicken 24

    Keto Lectin-Free Meatloaf 25

    Shrimp and Avocado Salad 26

Kale Salad 27

Easy Sardine Salad 28

Skillet Beef and Cabbage Stir Fry 29

Puerto Rican Beef and Onions 30

Lemon Garlic Salmon 31

Keto Lectin-Free Salmon Curry 32

Cauliflower and Broccoli Tuna Bowl 33

Keto Lectin-Free Beef and Spinach Quiche 34

Easy Chicken Hash 35

Crockpot Pesto Chicken Breast 36

Dill Tuna Salad 37

Chicken and Egg Salad Stuffed Avocado 38

Dinner Recipes 39

Grilled Chicken Skewers with Garlic Sauce 39

Baked Halibut with Lemon 40

Easy Coconut Chicken 41

Garlic Butter Chicken 42

Roasted Cilantro Chicken Thighs 43

Stir-Fried Ground Beef with Napa Cabbage 44

Broccoli Beef Stir Fry 45

Mustard, Cucumber, And Sardines Salad 46

Garlic Pan-Fried Cod 47

Lettuce Beef Wraps 48

Keto Lectin-Free Salmon Patties 49

Oven-Fried Breaded Broccoli Bites 50

Pork Adobo 51

Simple Chicken Egg Soup 52

Tuna Fish Salad 53

Snacks Recipes 54

Macaroon Fat Bombs 54

Mint Popsicles with Micro Greens 55

Coconut Boosters 56

Keto Lectin-Free Coffee 57

Indian Samosas 58

Stuffed Mushrooms 60

Hard Boiled Eggs 61

Pork Rinds Chicharron 62

Fried Seaweed Snack 63

Keto Lectin-Free Guacamole 64

Keto Lectin-Free Taco Meat 65

Brussels Sprouts Chips 66

Avocado Dip 67

Keto Lectin-Free Fat Balls 68

Steak Bites 69

Introduction

Losing weight but having so many health issues can be difficult. The thing is, there is no one-size-fits-all diet regimen to answer all your needs. In most cases, you have to do due diligence in order to find out how you can tweak a particular diet regimen so that you can get the most out of it and would fit your new lifestyle.

For instance, if you have been wondering why you still don't lose weight on a ketogenic diet despite following the guidelines strictly, then there must be something wrong with your body that prevents you from achieving your goals. Studies show that people who have damaged guts have the inability to properly absorb nutrients and also metabolize fats. This is the reason why even if you are diligently following the ketogenic diet, you are still unable to see any good results.

Thus, before you aim at weight loss, you need to focus more on healing your body by eating the right foods. This is where the lectin-free diet comes in. Lectin, a special protein found in many plants, is used by plants as part of their defenses against herbivory. These proteins are found provoke the inflammatory responses within the stomach.

People naturally react to lectin, but our reaction varies from one person to the other. Thus, the lectin-free diet is aimed at reducing the body's inflammatory responses so that we don't develop a leaky gut. While your focus is to heal your body first before weight loss, would it best if you can combine both the ketogenic and lectin-free diet so that you don't only heal your gut, but you also lose weight at the same time? Thus, this is where this hybrid diet regimen comes in. As a hybrid diet program, there are not too many information available about the keto lectin-free diet thus this eBook.

Let this book serve as your guide on the keto lectin-free diet.

Understanding the Keto Lectin-Free Diet

While some people are successful in losing weight through the ketogenic diet, there are others who are not despite that they are strictly following the guidelines. You might be one of the few people who suffer from food sensitivities.

Research shows that few of the population suffer from sensitivities toward the food that they eat. This is the reason that despite stringently following guidelines, you might find yourself unable to achieve your weight loss goals.

While the ketogenic diet can help you lose weight, if you suffer from gut problems, you need to deal with it first before you even aim for weight loss. As such you need to do clean eating. There are so many types of diets that you follow to address your digestive issues but what pairs with the ketogenic diet well is the lectin-free diet.

Combining both the ketogenic and lectin-free diets will not only help you deal with your gut issues, but it also helps you lose weight at the same time thus you get to kill two birds with one stone at the same time with this hybrid diet program.

What Is the Keto Lectin-Free Diet

The keto lectin-free diet is a marriage between the ketogenic and lectin-free diet. It was developed to address the growing problem of people who suffer from digestive problems and want to lose weight. The reason why people successfully lose weight is not solely due to calorie restriction, but it has something to do with having a healthy digestive system.

If your digestive system is not in a whack, you will be able to absorb all nutrients into your body effectively so even if you are following a very restrictive diet, you don't deny your body with the nutrient it receives with what little variety of food that you ingest.

With this hybrid diet regimen, you will be able to address your health issues and, at the same time, enjoy the benefits of weight loss. In a nutshell, what this diet does is that it pushes your body in a state of ketosis so that you burn more fats off while it also clears your digestive system from its many issues, so you can absorb important nutrients while under a diet.

And since lectin is a protein that binds to carbohydrate molecules, combining it [lectin-free diet] with the ketogenic diet means that the lectin will have only a little amount of carbohydrates that it can bind to thus it is very beneficial to the body.

Lastly, what makes the ketogenic and lectin-free diet a match made in heaven is that both diets almost have the same restrictions thus you can easily adjust the ingredients when making meals.

Keto Lectin-Free Diet Guidelines

When following this particular diet regimen, it is important that you follow important guidelines so that you will be able to achieve your health goals. Since the keto lectin-free diet is a combination of two popular diets, there are several things that you need to strictly follow before you can see any results.

- Avoid all foods that are high in lectin. A list of which foods to eat and avoid will be discussed in the next sections.
- Cook your food thoroughly to destroy lectin. While most plant ingredients contain lectin, they are easily destroyed with high heat.
- Fermented or sprouted legumes or grains to reduce their lectin content.
- Consume more fat than protein and make sure that you consume healthy fats.
- Plan your meals ahead so that you don't consume foods that are not allowed for both diets.

Food That You Can Consume

The ketogenic diet encourages you to consume more fats, moderate amounts of protein, and a small fraction of carbohydrates to jumpstart the state of ketosis in the body. On the other hand, the lectin-free diet is all about avoiding lectin that binds to carbohydrates thus making it more difficult for you to lose weight especially if you consume too many carbohydrates. So, what can you eat while following this diet regimen? Read on below to find out.

- **Healthy fats:** It is important to take note that not all fats are created equal. For this particular diet, it is important to opt for healthy sources of fat such as olive oil, butter, MCT oil, and coconut oil. Avocado is allowed for both the lectin-free and ketogenic diet.

- **Fatty fish and seafood:** Fatty fishes are a great source of healthy fats such as Omega-3s. You can source them from sardines, trout, salmon, and most fishes. Aside from fish, other seafood that you can consume include shrimps, lobsters, and shellfish as long as they are wild-caught.

- **Meats:** Animal proteins are allowed for this particular diet. Source them from pork, beef, chicken, turkey, and organ meats. However, stick to only a matchbox-sized portion so that you don't get kicked out of ketosis.

- **Eggs:** Eggs are allowed for both the ketogenic and lectin-free diet. It is a good source of healthy fats as well as protein.

- **Berries:** Berries such as strawberries, cherries, and blueberries are allowed for this diet. Not only do they contain low amounts of lectin, but they also contain a lot of antioxidants that are great for the body.

- **Grain-Free Flour Alternatives:** There are other grain-free flour alternatives that you can use when following the keto lectin-free diet and one of the best alternatives is the coconut flour. Technically, coconut is not really a nut but part of the drupe family. Other flours that are included but should be consumed in moderation include almond flour and hazelnut flour.

- **Citrus:** Citrus fruits such as lemon, lime, and oranges are allowed for both diet regimen.

- **Vegetables:** Vegetables especially grown above the ground are allowed for both the lectin and the ketogenic diet. Examples of vegetables that you can consume include broccoli, cauliflower, asparagus, and other green leafy vegetables.

- **Mozzarella cheese:** While most dairy products contain lectin, mozzarella cheese is an exception.

- **Sweeteners:** Sweeteners usually contain high amounts of carbohydrates but while it is accepted in the lectin-free diet, it is not allowed in the ketogenic diet. However, acceptable types of sweeteners include stevia and erythritol because both have a low glycemic index.

- **Water:** Water is technically not food, but it is the most acceptable beverage for both diet regimens as they don't contain any calories or anything that can drive the inflammatory processes in the body. Other beverages that are allowed are tea and coffee.

Food to Avoid

Both the lectin-free and ketogenic diet are highly restrictive when it comes to the types of foods that you are allowed to consume. This is to ensure that the food that you eat will not kick you out of ketosis but will also not cause any problems with your digestive system. Thus, below are the types of foods that you should avoid while following the keto lectin-free diet.

- **All vegetables from the nightshade family:** Plants belonging to the nightshade family are known to contain compounds that can drive the inflammatory responses in the body. Moreover, they also contain high amounts of lectin. Vegetables that belong to the nightshade family include tomatoes, eggplant, peppers, potatoes, and goji berries. Avoid them at all cost even if they are allowed in the ketogenic diet. Aside from vegetables belonging to the nightshade family, it is also important to avoid vegetables such as pumpkin and squash because they contain high amounts of lectin.

- **All legumes:** Legumes are not allowed in the ketogenic diet because they contain high amounts of starch that can kick out of ketosis. But more than carbohydrates, legumes also contain high amounts of lectin thus it is not allowed in the lectin-free diet. Stay away from all forms of beans such as peanuts, chickpeas, mung beans, kidney beans, and basically all beans imaginable.

- **All peanut-based products:** Peanut is a type of legume that contains high amounts of lectin. But it is not only peanuts that you should avoid but literally all ingredients that contain peanuts such as peanut butter and peanut oil.

- **All grains:** Grains are already not allowed in the ketogenic diet because it contains high amounts of carbohydrates. But didn't you know that it also contains high amounts of lectin? Avoid all types of grains such as rice, wheat, rye, sorghum, and many others. Moreover, it is also important to avoid products that are made from grain such as cakes, bread, and crackers.

- **All dairy products:** Dairy products contain high amounts of lectin. Avoid consuming milk, cream, and cheese. But if you cannot live without dairy, there is still a way for you to consume dairy products under this diet as long as the milk and milk products are pasteurized. Pasteurization destroys the lectin thereby neutralizing its amount to a lower degree.

- **Root crops:** Some root crops such as carrots and turnips contain low amounts of lectin but since they contain high amounts of carbohydrates, they should not be consumed while following the keto lectin-free diet.

- **Meat from corn-fed animals:** While meat is allowed in the keto lectin-free diet, it is important to avoid those that are sourced from corn-fed animals. Animals that are raised in conventional and modern husbandry methods are usually fed with grains. The lectin from the grain feed makes it to the entire system of the animal. This affects the quality of the meat obtained from the animal once slaughtered. Make sure that your meat is pasture-raised as they only eat natural grass or foods that they would naturally consume in the wild. This tip also holds true when buying fish. Make sure that you opt for wild-caught fish instead of farm-raised because they [farm-raised] are fed grains.

- **Nuts and seeds:** Nuts and seeds might be good snack options for dieters following the ketogenic diet. But since they contain high amounts of lectin, they should be avoided in the keto-lectin diet. Examples of nuts and seeds that should be avoided include chia seeds, almonds, walnuts, and sesame seeds.

- **Sugar:** Free sugar such as maple syrup, honey, brown sugar, molasses, white sugar, and fruit sugars contain high glycemic index thus it can kick the fat metabolism out. As such avoid anything that contains sugar such as soda and fruit juices.

- **Processed oils:** Processed oils are discouraged in the ketogenic diet but more importantly, they might be sourced from ingredients that contain high amounts of lectin such as soy and corn. Examples of processed oils that should be avoided include soy oil, corn oil, and canola oil.

- **Yeast:** Yeast contains certain amounts of lectin that can cause inflammation within the digestive tract. Avoid products that contain yeast including bread, wine, beer, and other fermented foods.

The Benefits of The Keto Lectin-Free Diet

This keto lectin-free diet regimen may sound too restrictive but there are so many benefits that you can get from combining the two. Below are the benefits and reasons why you need to try this diet regimen especially if each separate diet regimens are not effective separately.

- **Clear your food sensitivities:** Lectin binds to the cell membranes of the digestive tract thus it disrupts the metabolism and eventually causing damage to the gut such as the leaky gut. If you are prone to suffering from gastrointestinal problems, then avoiding lectin can help you clear your digestive tract from any food sensitivities. It can also improve the fat-burning ability of your body.

- **Help you avoid eating potentially toxic food:** Lectin can be toxic to the body especially if consumed in large amounts. By opting for the keto lectin-free diet, you will be able to avoid eating foods that are potentially toxic.

- **Lose weight healthily:** Perhaps the best thing about this particular diet regimen is that you can lose weight in a healthy way. Since your digestive issues are cleared with this regimen, your gut is still able to absorb the necessary nutrients to drive the physiologic functions of your body.

- **Easy to follow:** Despite its many restrictions, the keto lectin-free diet is very easy to follow. You can make recipes despite that there are several ingredients that you can use. All it takes is to use your creativity in the kitchen or follow the ingredients in this eBook.

The keto lectin free diet might sound too restrictive for most people, but you can still create very delicious meals that will not only help you lose weight but will also protect your digestive system from any inflammatory responses. With this diet regimen, you will be able to kill two birds with one stone.

Breakfast Recipes

Avocado Smoothie

Serves: 1
Cooking Time: 3 minutes

Ingredients
- ½ ripe avocado
- ½ cup coconut milk
- 1 handful of greens (spinach, kale or whatever is available)
- 1 cup ice
- 2 tablespoons liquid stevia

Instructions
1. Place all ingredients in the blender.
2. Pulse until all ingredients is smooth.
3. Serve immediately.

Nutrition information: Calories per serving:791; Carbohydrates: 23.2g; Protein: 9.7g; Fat:86.9 g; Fiber: 15.2g

Breakfast Burger with Avocado

Serves: 1

Cooking Time: 15 minutes

Ingredients
- 2 bacon strips
- 1 egg
- 1 ripe avocado
- 1 slice red onion
- 1 lettuce leaf
- Salt and pepper to taste

Instructions
1. Heat the frying pan over medium flame. Fry the bacon until crispy and the fat has rendered. Set aside.
2. Using the same pan with the rendered bacon fat, crack the egg and use bacon fat to cook the egg until the yolk is no longer runny. Set aside.
3. Slice the avocado in half and remove the pit. Peel the avocado so that it resembles a burger bun.
4. Assemble the burger by layering one avocado "bun", onion, lettuce, bacon, and egg. Season with salt and pepper and top with the remaining avocado bun.
5. Serve.

Nutrition information: Calories per serving:504; Carbohydrates: 13.2g; Protein:20.5 g; Fat: 54.9g; Fiber: 9.3g

Cauliflower and Ground Beef Skillet

Serves: 4
Cooking Time: 20 minutes

Ingredients
- 2 tablespoons ghee
- ½ small onion, chopped
- 2 cloves of garlic, minced
- 1-pound ground beef
- Salt and pepper to taste
- ½ cup water
- 1 small head cauliflower, sliced thinly
- 1 tablespoon coconut aminos
- 4 large eggs
- ½ ripe avocado, flesh scooped
- 1 tablespoon parsley, chopped

Instructions
1. Preheat the oven to 350°F.
2. In a skillet, heat the ghee over medium flame and sauté the onion and garlic for 1 minute. Stir in the ground beef and season with salt and pepper to taste.
3. Add water. Cover and allow to simmer for 7 minutes.
4. Stir in the cauliflower and season with coconut aminos.
5. Make four depressions in the mixture and crack in the eggs.
6. Place the skillet in the oven and broil for 10 minutes.
7. Once the eggs are cooked, garnish with avocado slices and parsley.

Nutrition information: Calories per serving: 454; Carbohydrates: 8.1g; Protein: 38g; Fat: 52.4g; Fiber: 6.6g

Avocado Salmon Breakfast Cups

Serves: 1

Cooking Time: 5 minutes

Ingredients
- 1 ripe avocado
- 2 ounces wild-caught salmon, smoked and flaked
- 2 tablespoons extra virgin olive oil
- Juice from 1 lemon
- Salt to taste

Instructions
1. Cut the avocado in half and remove the seed.
2. In a mixing bowl, place the rest of the ingredients and mix until well-combined.
3. Scoop the salmon mixture into the avocado (where the seed once was).
4. Serve.

Nutrition information: Calories per serving: 525; Carbohydrates: 4g; Protein: 19g; Fat: 48g; Fiber: 1.2g

Cauliflower Fritters

Serves: 6
Cooking Time: 15 minutes

Ingredients
- 1 large cauliflower head, broken into florets
- 2 eggs, beaten
- ½ teaspoon turmeric
- ½ teaspoon salt
- ¼ teaspoon black pepper
- 6 tablespoons ghee

Instructions
1. Place the cauliflower florets in a pot with water. Bring to a boil for 6 minutes.
2. Once cooked, drain and Addto food processor.
3. Place the eggs, turmeric, salt, and pepper into the food processor.
4. Pulse until the mixture becomes coarse.
5. Transfer into a bowl. Using your hands, form six small flattened balls and place in the fridge for at least 1 hour until the mixture hardens.
6. Heat the oil in a skillet and fry the cauliflower patties for 3 minutes on each side

Nutrition information: Calories per serving:157; Carbohydrates: 2.8g; Protein: 3.9g; Fat: 15.3g; Fiber:0.9 g

Coconut Flour Porridge

Serves: 1

Cooking Time: 5 minutes

Ingredients
- 2 tablespoons coconut flour
- 2 tablespoons golden flax meal
- ¾ cup water
- A pinch of salt
- 1 egg, beaten
- 2 teaspoons ghee
- 3 tablespoons coconut milk
- Berries for topping

Instructions
1. In a saucepan, place the first four ingredients and bring to a simmer.
2. Remove from the heat and add the beaten egg while stirring constantly.
3. Turn on the heat and whisk until the mixture thickens.
4. Add the ghee and coconut milk.
5. Pour in a bowl and allow to cool completely before garnishing with berries of your choice.

Nutrition information: Calories per serving: 453; Carbohydrates: 14g; Protein: 13g; Fat: 39g; Fiber:3 g

Avocado Smoothie with Coconut Milk, Ginger, And Turmeric

Serves: 1
Cooking Time: 3 minutes

Ingredients

- ½ avocado, pitted and flesh scooped out
- ¾ cup coconut milk
- ¼ cup almond milk
- 1 teaspoon ginger, grated
- ½ teaspoon turmeric powder
- 1 cup crushed ice
- 1 tablespoon stevia powder

Instructions

1. Add all ingredients in the blender.
2. Blend on low speed until everything is smooth.
3. Serve immediately.

Nutrition information: Calories per serving: 208; Carbohydrates: 5g; Protein: 1g; Fat: 21g; Fiber: 1g

Shrimp Omelet

Serves: 2

Cooking Time: 7 minutes

Ingredients

- 3 tablespoons olive oil
- ¼ onion, chopped
- 10 large shrimps, peeled and deveined
- 6 eggs, beaten
- 1 handful of spinach, shredded

Instructions

1. Heat oil in a skillet over medium flame.
2. Sauté the onion for 1 minute until fragrant.
3. Add the shrimps and stir for 30 seconds.
4. Pour in the eggs and top with spinach.
5. Adjust the flame to low and cover the skillet with a lid.
6. Allow to cook for 6 minutes or until the eggs are set.
7. Serve warm.

Nutrition information: Calories per serving:329; Carbohydrates: 4g; Protein: 17g; Fat: 36g; Fiber: 0.4g

Steak and Eggs

Serves: 1
Cooking Time: 10 minutes

Ingredients
- 1 tablespoon ghee
- 3 eggs
- Salt and pepper to taste
- 4-ounce sirloin steak
- ¼ avocado

Instructions
1. Heat ghee in a skillet over medium flame and cook the eggs sunny side up for 2 minutes on each side. Season with salt and pepper to taste. Set aside.
2. Using the same pan, sear the sirloin to the desired doneness. Slice into strips and season with salt and pepper.
3. Serve the sirloin strips with eggs and avocado.

Nutrition information: Calories per serving: 510; Carbohydrates: 3g; Protein: 26g; Fat: 44g; Fiber: 0.9g

Guacamole Eggs

Serves: 3

Cooking Time: 3 minutes

Ingredients

- 6 hardboiled eggs, cooled and peeled
- 1 teaspoon garlic, minced
- 1 teaspoon shallot, minced
- 1 avocado, pitted and meat scooped out
- 1 teaspoon lemon juice
- Salt and pepper to taste
- 3 tablespoons fried bacon bits

Instructions

1. Place eggs in a mixing bowl and mash.
2. Add the garlic, shallots, and avocado.
3. Mix while mashing at the same time to incorporate all ingredients.
4. Add the lemon juice and season with salt and pepper to taste.
5. Garnish with bacon bits on top.

Nutrition information: Calories per serving: 408; Carbohydrates: 11.7g; Protein: 21.9g; Fat: 30.9g; Fiber: 6.2g

Bacon and Basil Egg Omelet

Serves: 2
Cooking Time: 8 minutes

Ingredients
- 2 tablespoons olive oil
- 2 strips of bacon
- 2 cloves of garlic minced
- ½ cup basil leaves
- 3 eggs, beaten
- Salt and pepper to taste

Instructions
1. Heat oil in a skillet dish over medium flame.
2. Fry the bacon on both sides until crispy. Crumble then set aside.
3. Using the same pan, sauté the garlic and basil leaves for 30 seconds.
4. Pour in the eggs. Season with salt and pepper.
5. Cook on both sides for 3 minutes each.

Nutrition information: Calories per serving: 343; Carbohydrates: 4.9g; Protein: 14.6g; Fat: 29.5g; Fiber: 2.3g

Keto Strawberry Breakfast Smoothie

Serves: 1

Cooking Time: 3 minutes

Ingredients
- 1 cup coconut milk
- ½ cup organic strawberries
- ½ teaspoon cinnamon powder
- ½ cup crushed ice

Instructions
1. Place all ingredients in a blender.
2. Blend until smooth.
3. Serve chilled.

Nutrition information: Calories per serving: 721; Carbohydrates: 12.1g; Protein: 28.3g; Fat: 65.8g; Fiber: 7.3g

Breakfast Sausage Casserole

Serves: 10
Cooking Time: 10 minutes

Ingredients
- 3 tablespoons avocado oil
- 1-pound sausage without casing
- 2 cloves of garlic, minced
- ½ teaspoon chopped onion
- ¼ cup chopped broccoli
- 12 eggs, beaten
- ½ cup coconut milk
- Salt and pepper to taste

Instructions
1. Heat the oil in a casserole dish and sauté the sausage, garlic, and onions. Keep stirring for 2 minutes.
2. Stir in the broccoli, eggs, and coconut milk. Season with salt and pepper to taste.
3. Cover the casserole with the lid and adjust the heat to low.
4. Cook for 6 to 10 minutes until the eggs are set.
5. Serve warm.

Nutrition information: Calories per serving: 276; Carbohydrates: 5.2g; Protein: 17.9g; Fat: 25.8g; Fiber: 1.9g

Coconut Cherry Vanilla Smoothie

Serves: 1

Cooking Time: 3 minutes

Ingredients
- 2 ½ ounces full fat coconut milk
- 3 ½ ounces filtered water
- 1/8 teaspoon pure vanilla essence
- A pinch of salt
- 3 ounces organic cherries
- 8 ice cubes

Instructions
1. Place all ingredients in the blender.
2. Pulse until smooth.
3. Serve chilled.

Nutrition information: Calories per serving: 218; Carbohydrates: 7.6g; Protein: 2.4g; Fat: 27.1g; Fiber: 4.6g

Bacon Spinach Frittata

Serves: 8
Cooking Time: 20 minutes

Ingredients
- 8 large eggs, beaten
- 4 large egg whites, beaten
- 1 cup coconut milk
- ¼ cup onion, diced
- 2 cups spinach
- 6 bacon strips, fried and crumbled

Instructions
1. Preheat the oven to 400 degrees.
2. In a heat-proof dish, place all ingredients and give a good whisk.
3. Place inside the oven and cook for 20 minutes or until the eggs are cooked through.

Nutrition information: Calories per serving:147; Carbohydrates: 3.2g; Protein: 5.8g; Fat: 12.8g; Fiber: 1.6g

Lunch Recipes

Lemon Balsamic Chicken

Serves: 6

Cooking Time: 30 minutes

Ingredients
- 5 tablespoons olive oil
- 3 tablespoons butter, grass-fed
- 8 boneless chicken thighs
- 1 cup sliced onion
- 2 tablespoons minced lemon rind
- 2 bay leaves
- 1 teaspoon dried Italian herb blend
- 1 ½ tablespoons balsamic vinegar
- Salt and pepper to taste

Instructions
1. In a large skillet, heat the oil and butter and sear the chicken thighs for 3 minutes on each side.
2. Add the onion, lemon rind, bay leaves, Italian herb, balsamic vinegar, salt and pepper.
3. Adjust the moisture by adding a cup of water.
4. Close the lid and continue cooking for 25 minutes.
5. Open the lid and allow the sauce to simmer and thicken.

Nutrition information: Calories per serving:758; Carbohydrates: 18.5g; Protein: 33.5g; Fat: 68.1g; Fiber: 13.7g

Keto Lectin-Free Meatloaf

Serves: 10
Cooking Time: 50 minutes

Ingredients
- 2 pounds grass-fed ground beef
- ½ tablespoon salt
- 1 teaspoon black pepper
- 2 large eggs, beaten
- 2 tablespoons olive oil
- ¼ cup chopped parsley
- 4 cloves of garlic, minced

Instructions
1. Preheat the oven to 400^0F.
2. In a mixing bowl, combine all ingredients until all ingredients are well-combined.
3. Place in an 8x4 inches loaf pan and flatten the mixture with a spatula.
4. Set in the middle rack of the oven and cook for 50 minutes.
5. Once cooked, allow to cool before removing from the loaf pan.

Nutrition information: Calories per serving:344; Carbohydrates: 4g; Protein:28 g; Fat: 37g; Fiber: 2g

Shrimp and Avocado Salad

Serves: 2

Cooking Time: 5 minutes

Ingredients

- ½ pound large shrimps, peeled and deveined
- 2 cloves of garlic, minced
- 1 teaspoon ground basil
- 1 teaspoon dried thyme
- Salt and pepper to taste
- 1 teaspoon olive oil
- 4 cups Cos lettuce leaves
- 1 avocado, pitted and cubed
- ¼ red onion, sliced
- Juice from 1 lemon

Instructions

1. In a mixing bowl, combine the shrimps, garlic, ground basil, and thyme. Season with salt and pepper to taste.
2. Heat oil in a skillet and sauté the shrimps until cooked. Set aside.
3. Assemble the salad by combining the lettuce leaves, avocado, and onion. Toss in the shrimps.
4. Season with lemon juice, salt and pepper.
5. Toss to combine everything.

Nutrition information: Calories per serving:235; Carbohydrates: 3.5g; Protein:4.8 g; Fat: 17.4g; Fiber: 1.8g

Kale Salad

Serves: 2
Cooking Time: 5 minutes

Ingredients
- 2 slices of fried bacon, diced
- 1 cooked chicken breast, diced
- 2 hardboiled egg, peeled and sliced
- 8 raspberries
- A large bag of kale leaves, chopped
- 3 tablespoons olive oil
- ½ teaspoon mustard
- 1 clove of garlic, minced
- Salt and pepper to taste

Instructions
1. In a mixing bowl, combine the bacon, chicken, egg, raspberries, and kale.
2. Toss to combine all ingredients.
3. In a small bowl, mix together olive oil, mustard, garlic, salt and pepper.
4. Drizzle over the salad. Toss to coat ingredients with the dressing.

Nutrition information: Calories per serving: 640; Carbohydrates: 7g; Protein: 38g; Fat: 51g; Fiber: 5g

Easy Sardine Salad

Serves: 1

Cooking Time: 5 minutes

Ingredients
- 1 can sardines in olive oil, drained
- ¼ pound salad greens
- ¼ cup leftover meat, chopped
- ¼ onion, chopped
- 1 tablespoon olive oil
- 1 tablespoon lemon juice
- Salt and pepper to taste

Instructions
1. In a salad bowl, combine the sardines, salad greens, leftover meat, and onion.
2. In a small mixing bowl, combine the olive oil, lemon juice, salt and pepper.
3. Drizzle the dressing onto the salad.
4. Toss to coat all ingredients.

Nutrition information: Calories per serving:400; Carbohydrates:2 g; Protein: 30g; Fat: 34g; Fiber: 0.8g

Skillet Beef and Cabbage Stir Fry

Serves: 5
Cooking Time: 15 minutes

Ingredients

- 1-pound uncured bacon, chopped
- 1-pound ground beef, grass-fed
- 1 onion, chopped
- 3 cloves of garlic, minced
- Salt and pepper to taste
- 1 head of cabbage, chopped

Instructions

1. In a large skillet, sauté the bacon until it has rendered fat and is crispy. Set aside.
2. In the same skillet, sauté the ground beef, onion, and garlic for 5 minutes.
3. Season with salt and pepper to taste.
4. Adjust the moisture by adding enough water.
5. Close the lid and allow to simmer for another 5 minutes.
6. Open the lid and stir in the cabbage.
7. Cook for another 5 minutes.

Nutrition information: Calories per serving: 357; Carbohydrates: 6.9g; Protein: 31g; Fat: 21.9g; Fiber: 2.5g

Puerto Rican Beef and Onions

Serves: 4

Cooking Time: 15 minutes

Ingredients
- 3 tablespoons lard
- 3 tablespoons olive oil
- 4 beef steaks, cubed
- Salt and pepper to taste
- 1 teaspoon coconut aminos
- 2 tablespoons coconut vinegar
- 2 white onion, sliced

Instructions
1. In a skillet over medium flame, heat the lard and olive oil.
2. Stir in the steak slices and season with salt, pepper, and coconut aminos.
3. Continue stirring for 5 minutes.
4. Add the vinegar.
5. Close the lid and adjust the flame to medium low.
6. Allow to simmer for 10 minutes.
7. Open the lid and Add the white onion. Cook for another 2 minutes.

Nutrition information: Calories per serving: 509; Carbohydrates: 1.1g; Protein: 23.1g; Fat: 58.1g; Fiber: 0g

Lemon Garlic Salmon

Serves: 2
Cooking Time: 10 minutes

Ingredients
- 2 filets of salmon, wild-caught
- 6 tablespoons ghee
- 4 cloves of garlic, minced
- 2 teaspoons lemon juice
- Salt and pepper to taste

Instructions
1. Mix all ingredients in a bowl.
2. Allow to marinate in the fridge for at least 2 hours.
3. Heat the grill to medium high and cook the salmon for 3 to 5 minutes on both sides.
4. Serve with grilled asparagus and slices of avocado.

Nutrition information: Calories per serving: 599; Carbohydrates: 2.1g; Protein: 26.8; Fat: 58.6g; Fiber:0.2g

Keto Lectin-Free Salmon Curry

Serves: 2

Cooking Time: 8 minutes

Ingredients
- 2 tablespoons coconut oil
- ½ onion, sliced
- 1 ½ tablespoons of curry powder
- 1 teaspoon garlic powder
- 2 cups coconut milk
- 1 pound wild-caught raw salmon, diced
- 2 tablespoon chopped basil

Instructions
1. In a deep pan, heat the coconut oil over medium heat and sauté the onion, curry powder and garlic powder until fragrant.
2. Add the coconut milk and salmon.
3. Close the lid and allow to simmer for 6 minutes.
4. Add chopped basil and cook for another minute.
5. Serve warm.

Nutrition information: Calories per serving: 640; Carbohydrates: 16g; Protein: 32g; Fat: 49g; Fiber: 6g

Cauliflower and Broccoli Tuna Bowl

Serves: 4
Cooking Time: 20 minutes

Ingredients

- 1 head cauliflower, cut into florets
- 1 head broccoli, cut into florets
- 2 tablespoons olive oil
- Juice from 1 lemon
- Salt to taste
- 3 tablespoons coconut aminos
- 4 cans of tuna in oil, drained
- 2 hard-boiled eggs, peeled and mashed

Instructions

1. Preheat the oven to 400^0F.
2. In a baking dish, place the cauliflower and broccoli and drizzle with olive oil, lemon, and salt.
3. Bake in the oven for 20 minutes.
4. Once slightly golden, remove from the oven.
5. Toss into a bowl and stir in coconut aminos, tuna, and eggs.
6. Mix to combine.

Nutrition information: Calories per serving: 435; Carbohydrates: 15g; Protein: 25g; Fat: 38g; Fiber: 7g

Keto Lectin-Free Beef and Spinach Quiche

Serves: 2

Cooking Time: 20 minutes

Ingredients
- 3 tablespoons olive oil
- 2 tablespoons ghee
- 3 cloves of garlic
- ½ pound ground beef, grass-fed
- Salt and pepper to taste
- 3 eggs, beaten
- ¼ cup coconut milk
- ¼ cup leek, chopped

Instructions
1. In a skillet, heat the oil and ghee and sauté the garlic and ground beef for 5 minutes until the beef is done. Season with salt and pepper to taste.
2. Transfer the beef in a heat-proof dish (meat and oil).
3. In a mixing bowl, combine eggs and coconut milk.
4. Pour over the sautéed ground beef and Add the leeks.
5. Season with more salt and pepper if desired.
6. Place in a 400°F preheated oven and cook for 15 minutes or until the eggs are cooked through.

Nutrition information: Calories per serving: 855; Carbohydrates: 3.1g; Protein: 24.8g; Fat: 71.2g; Fiber: 1.5g

Easy Chicken Hash

Serves: 6

Cooking Time:

Ingredients

- 4 tablespoons coconut oil
- 4 chicken breasts, sliced into small slices
- Salt and pepper to taste
- 1 onion, sliced thinly
- 1 leek sliced

Instructions

1. Place all ingredients in a crockpot.
2. Close the lid and cook on high for 4 hours.
3. Take the meat out and shred using two forks.
4. Serve with sauce.

Nutrition information: Calories per serving: 423; Carbohydrates: 2.9g; Protein: 27.1g; Fat: 40.7g; Fiber: 1.2g

Crockpot Pesto Chicken Breast

Serves: 2

Cooking Time: 4 hours

Ingredients
- ¼ cup olive oil
- 1 ½ cups basil leaves
- 2 cloves of garlic, chopped
- Juice from ½ lemon
- A dash of salt to taste
- 2 chicken breasts

Instructions
1. In a food processor, combine olive oil, basil leaves, garlic, and lemon juice. Pulse until smooth.
2. Place chicken in a crockpot and pour over the pesto sauce.
3. Close the crockpot and cook on high for 4 hours.

Nutrition information: Calories per serving: 745; Carbohydrates: 1.8g; Protein: 70.2g; Fat: 27.2g; Fiber: 0.4g

Dill Tuna Salad

Serves: 2

Cooking Time: 5 minutes

Ingredients
- 1 can tuna in oil, drained
- 3 tablespoons olive oil
- A pinch of fresh dill, chopped
- Salt and pepper to taste
- 1 avocado, pitted and meat scooped out

Instructions
1. In a mixing bowl, place all ingredients.
2. Toss to combine.
3. Chill before serving.

Nutrition information: Calories per serving: 514; Carbohydrates: 10.7g; Protein: 21.6g; Fat: 45.2g; Fiber: 5.3g

Chicken and Egg Salad Stuffed Avocado

Serves: 2

Cooking Time: 5 minutes

Ingredients
- 4 hardboiled eggs, peeled and diced
- 1 cup cooked chicken, shredded
- 3 tablespoons ghee
- 2 tablespoons parsley, chopped
- Salt and pepper to taste
- 1 avocado

Instructions
1. In a mixing bowl, combine the eggs, chicken, ghee, and parsley. Season with salt and pepper to taste.
2. Slice the avocado lengthwise and remove the pit or seed.
3. Scoop the egg and chicken mixture and place in the avocado (where the seed once was).
4. Chill before serving.

Nutrition information: Calories per serving:837; Carbohydrates: 12.9g; Protein: 28.1g; Fat: 74.1g; Fiber: 6.2g

Dinner Recipes

Grilled Chicken Skewers with Garlic Sauce

Serves: 2
Cooking Time: 10 minutes

Ingredients
- 1-pound chicken breast, cut into large cubes
- 1 onion, wedged
- 2 tablespoons olive oil
- Salt and pepper to taste
- 1 head garlic, peeled
- 1 teaspoon salt
- ¼ cup lemon juice
- 1 cup olive oil

Instructions
1. Preheat the grill to medium high.
2. Skewer the chicken breast and onions on a bamboo or metal skewer.
3. Brush with olive oil and season with salt and pepper to taste.
4. Grill for 3 to 5 minutes on each side.
5. While the chicken is grilling, grill the garlic for 10 minutes.
6. Peel off the garlic skin and place in a food processor together with salt, lemon juice and oil.
7. Blend until well combined.
8. Serve the chicken with the garlic sauce.

Nutrition information: Calories per serving: 1502; Carbohydrates: 3.7g; Protein: 48.4g; Fat: 142.6g; Fiber: 1.1g

Baked Halibut with Lemon

Serves: 4

Cooking Time: 10 minutes

Ingredients
- 2 11-ounce halibut steaks
- Juice from ½ lemon
- 1 teaspoon lemon zest, grated
- Salt and pepper to taste
- 4 tablespoons olive oil, divided

Instructions
1. In a bowl, combine the halibut steak, lemon juice, zest, salt, and pepper. Drizzle 1 tablespoon of the oil.
2. Allow to marinate in the fridge for at least 30 minutes.
3. Preheat the grill to medium high.
4. Grill the halibut steaks for 5 minutes on each side.
5. Before serving, drizzle with the remaining olive oil.

Nutrition information: Calories per serving:542; Carbohydrates: 1.6g; Protein: 39.4g; Fat: 41.2g; Fiber: 0.2g

Easy Coconut Chicken

Serves: 4
Cooking Time: 15 minutes

Ingredients
- 3 tablespoons coconut oil
- 5 cloves of garlic, peeled and crushed
- 1-pound boneless, skinless chicken thighs
- 4 tablespoons apple cider vinegar
- Salt and pepper to taste
- ¼ cup water
- 8-ounce coconut milk

Instructions
1. In a deep pan, heat the oil over medium high flame and sauté the garlic until fragrant. Stir in the chicken and sear all sides for at least 3 minutes.
2. Add the rest of the ingredients.
3. Close the lid and allow to boil.
4. Reduce the heat to medium and allow to simmer for 10 minutes.

Nutrition information: Calories per serving: 421; Carbohydrates: 4.0g; Protein: 29.0g; Fat: 32.7g; Fiber: 0.2g

Garlic Butter Chicken

Serves: 4

Cooking Time: 20 minutes

Ingredients
- 4 chicken breasts
- ¼ cup ghee
- 1 teaspoon turmeric
- 1 teaspoon salt
- 1/8 cup water
- 10 cloves of garlic, peeled and chopped

Instructions
1. Place all ingredients in a skillet and heat over medium flame.
2. Close the lid and allow to cook in its own natural juices for 15 minutes.
3. Open the lid and allow to simmer until the sauce thickens.

Nutrition information: Calories per serving: 404; Carbohydrates: 1 g; Protein: 28g; Fat: 51g; Fiber: 0.4g

Roasted Cilantro Chicken Thighs

Serves: 8
Cooking Time: 10 minutes

Ingredients
- 2 pounds boneless chicken thighs
- 4 tablespoons organic extra virgin olive oil
- Salt and pepper to taste
- 2 tablespoons chopped cilantro
- Juice from 1 lime

Instructions
1. Place all ingredients in a Ziploc bag and allow to marinate for at least 2 hours in the fridge.
2. Preheat the grill to medium for 10 minutes.
3. Grill the chicken for at least 5 minutes on each side.
4. Baste the chicken with the marinade.
5. Serve warm.

Nutrition information: Calories per serving: 410; Carbohydrates: 7.1g; Protein: 15.3g; Fat: 39.4g; Fiber: 4.3g

Stir-Fried Ground Beef with Napa Cabbage

Serves: 8

Cooking Time: 15 minutes

Ingredients

- 5 tablespoons lard
- 2 pounds grass-fed ground beef
- 4 cloves of garlic
- 1 onion, chopped
- 1 tablespoon grated ginger root
- ¾ cup coconut aminos
- ¼ cup water
- 1 head Napa cabbage
- Salt and pepper to taste

Instructions

1. In a skillet, heat oil over medium flame and stir in the ground beef, garlic, and onion for 3 minutes.
2. Pour in coconut aminos and water. Close the lid and allow to simmer for 10 minutes.
3. Open the lid and stir in the Napa cabbage.
4. Season with more salt and pepper to taste.
5. Close the lid and continue cooking for 2 minutes.

Nutrition information: Calories per serving:374; Carbohydrates: 3.2g; Protein: 16.4g; Fat: 37.2g; Fiber: 1.4g

Broccoli Beef Stir Fry

Serves: 2
Cooking Time: 15 minutes

Ingredients
- 4 tablespoons olive oil
- 3 cloves of garlic, peeled and chipped
- 1 teaspoon grated ginger
- ½ pound beef steak, sliced thinly
- 2 tablespoons coconut aminos
- 2 cups broccoli florets

Instructions
1. In a skillet, heat the olive oil over medium flame and sauté the garlic and ginger for 30 seconds.
2. Stir in the sliced beef and cook for 3 minutes. Season with coconut aminos.
3. Adjust the moisture by adding water.
4. Close the lid and allow to simmer for 10 minutes.
5. Open the lid and stir in the broccoli florets.
6. Cook for another 2 minutes.

Nutrition information: Calories per serving: 416; Carbohydrates: 3.3g; Protein: 15.4g; Fat: 44.7g; Fiber: 1.2g

Mustard, Cucumber, And Sardines Salad

Serves: 1
Cooking Time: 5 minutes

Ingredients
- 1 can sardines in olive oil, drained
- ¼ cup cucumber, peeled and diced
- 1 tablespoon lemon juice
- ½ tablespoon mustard
- 3 tablespoons olive oil
- Salt and pepper to taste

Instructions
1. In a bowl, combine all ingredients until well combined.
2. Allow to chill in the fridge before serving.

Nutrition information: Calories per serving:260; Carbohydrates: 2g; Protein: 17g; Fat: 30g; Fiber: 0.2g

Garlic Pan-Fried Cod

Serves: 4

Cooking Time: 7 minutes

Ingredients
- 4 tablespoons ghee
- 6 cloves of garlic, minced
- 4 cod filets
- Salt and pepper to taste

Instructions
1. In a skillet, heat the oil over medium flame and sauté the garlic until fragrant.
2. Pan fry the cod fillets for 3 minutes on each side. Season with salt and pepper to taste.
3. Serve warm.

Nutrition information: Calories per serving: 192; Carbohydrates: 1.5g; Protein: 12.5g; Fat: 24.2g; Fiber: 0.7g

Lettuce Beef Wraps

Serves: 8

Cooking Time: 13 minutes

Ingredients

- 5 tablespoons coconut oil
- ¼ onion, diced
- 4 cloves of garlic, minced
- ½ pound ground beef
- 1 teaspoon grated ginger
- 2 teaspoon cumin
- Salt and pepper to taste
- 2 tablespoons chopped cilantro
- 8 large lettuce leaves

Instructions

1. In a skillet, heat oil over medium flame and sauté the onion and garlic until fragrant.
2. Stir in the ground beef and continue stirring for 3 minutes.
3. Add the ginger, cumin, salt and pepper. Adjust the moisture by adding water.
4. Close the lid and allow to simmer for 10 minutes.
5. Turn off the heat and stir in the cilantro.
6. Allow to cool.
7. Serve with lettuce leaves.

Nutrition information: Calories per serving: 259; Carbohydrates:8.4 g; Protein: 12.3g; Fat: 27.1g; Fiber: 4.3g

Keto Lectin-Free Salmon Patties

Serves: 4

Cooking Time: 10 minutes

Ingredients
- ¼ pound smoked salmon, flaked
- 3 eggs, beaten
- ½ cup coconut flour
- 2 tablespoons chopped parsley
- 1 teaspoon chopped dill
- 1 tablespoon lemon juice
- ½ teaspoon turmeric
- 1 clove of garlic, chopped
- Salt and pepper to taste
- ½ cup coconut oil
- 1 small avocado, pitted and meat scooped out

Instructions
1. In a mixing bowl, combine all ingredients except for the coconut oil and avocado.
2. Mix to combine everything. Using your hands, form large patties with the mixture and set aside.
3. Heat oil in a skillet over medium flame. Once hot, fry the salmon patties until golden brown.
4. Place in a plate lined with paper towel to absorb the extra fat.
5. Serve with slices of avocado.

Nutrition information: Calories per serving:471; Carbohydrates: 8.4g; Protein: 14.2g; Fat: 44.1g; Fiber: 5.2g

Oven-Fried Breaded Broccoli Bites

Serves: 3

Cooking Time: 20 minutes

Ingredients
- 12 broccoli florets
- 1/3 cup coconut flour
- 1 teaspoon garlic powder
- ½ teaspoon salt
- ¼ teaspoon dried parsley
- 1 tablespoons mozzarella cheese, grated
- 2 eggs, beaten
- 2 tablespoons butter, melted
- 1 tablespoon olive oil

Instructions
1. In a Ziploc bag, combine all ingredients and give a good shake to coat the broccoli with the flour mixture.
2. Preheat the oven to 400°F.
3. Place the broccoli in a baking pan and cook in the oven for 20 minutes until crispy.

Nutrition information: Calories per serving:259; Carbohydrates: 4.1g; Protein: 18.8 Fat: 36.1g; Fiber: 2.8g

Pork Adobo

Serves: 4
Cooking Time: 20 minutes

Ingredients
- 3 tablespoons coconut oil
- 1 onion, sliced
- 4 cloves of garlic, minced
- 1-pound pork sirloin, cubed
- 3 tablespoons coconut aminos
- 2 tablespoon apple cider vinegar
- ¼ cup water
- 1 bay leaf
- Salt and pepper to taste
- 2 hardboiled eggs, peeled

Instructions
1. In a skillet, heat the oil over medium flame and sauté the onion and garlic until fragrant.
2. Stir in the pork and pan sear all edges.
3. Add the coconut aminos, apple cider vinegar, and water. Stir in the bay leaf and season with more salt and pepper to taste.
4. Close the lid and allow to simmer for 20 minutes.
5. A minute before the cooking time ends, add the hardboiled eggs.

Nutrition information: Calories per serving:296; Carbohydrates: 4.1g; Protein: 17.2g; Fat: 35.1g; Fiber: 3.1g

Simple Chicken Egg Soup

Serves: 4

Cooking Time: 6 minutes

Ingredients
- 3 tablespoons ghee or butter
- 2 tablespoons olive oil
- 1 onion, chopped
- 3 cloves of garlic, minced
- 1-pound chicken breasts, pre-cooked and shredded
- 3 cups water
- 1 teaspoon basil
- 1 teaspoon chopped parsley
- Salt and pepper to taste
- 3 eggs, beaten

Instructions
1. Heat the ghee and olive oil in a pan over medium flame and sauté the onion and garlic for 30 seconds.
2. Add the rest of the ingredients except for the eggs.
3. Bring water to a boil and allow to simmer for 6 minutes.
4. Pour over the beaten egg while stirring constantly.

Nutrition information: Calories per serving:440; Carbohydrates: 5.2g; Protein: 26.8g; Fat: 42.7g; Fiber: 3.9g

Tuna Fish Salad

Serves: 3

Cooking Time: 3 minutes

Ingredients

- 2 cups mixed greens
- ¼ cup parsley, chopped
- ¼ cup fresh mint, chopped
- 10 large kalamata olives, pitted and sliced
- ½ avocado, pitted and sliced
- 1 green onion, sliced
- 1 can tuna in oil, drained
- 3 tablespoons extra virgin olive oil
- 1 tablespoon balsamic vinegar
- Salt and pepper to taste

Instructions

1. Toss all ingredients in a salad bowl.
2. Mix until well-combined.
3. Place in the fridge to chill before serving.

Nutrition information: Calories per serving: 280; Carbohydrates: 3.6g; Protein: 20.9g; Fat: 38.2g; Fiber: 2.2g

Snacks Recipes

Macaroon Fat Bombs

Serves: 10
Cooking Time: 8 minutes

Ingredients
- ¼ cup coconut flour
- ½ cup shredded coconut
- 2 tablespoons powdered stevia
- 2 tablespoons coconut oil
- 3 egg whites, chilled

Instructions
1. In a mixing bowl, combine the coconut flour, shredded coconut and stevia. Set aside.
2. Melt the coconut oil in a saucepan and Addto the flour mixture. Blend until well-combined.
3. Put the egg whites in a chilled bowl and whisk until stiff. Incorporate the eggs into the flour mixture and fold.
4. Spoon the mixture into a baking sheet lined with parchment paper.
5. Bake in a 400^0F preheated oven for 8 minutes or until golden brown.

Nutrition information: Calories per serving: 46; Carbohydrates: 0.5g; Protein: 1.8g; Fat: 5g; Fiber: 0.2g

Mint Popsicles with Micro Greens

Serves: 4
Cooking Time: 5 minutes

Ingredients
- 1 can full fat coconut milk
- 2 cups fresh mint leaves, chopped
- 20 drops liquid stevia
- 1 cup micro greens
- A dash of cardamom

Instructions
1. Place all ingredients in a blender.
2. Pulse until smooth.
3. Pour into popsicle molds and freeze overnight to harden.

Nutrition information: Calories per serving: 159; Carbohydrates: 8.6g; Protein: 2.5g; Fat: 13g; Fiber: 3.2g

Coconut Boosters

Serves: 4
Cooking Time: 10 minutes

Ingredients
- 1 cup coconut oil
- ½ cup coconut flakes, unsweetened
- 1 teaspoon vanilla extract
- 3 eggs, beaten
- 20 drops liquid stevia

Instructions
1. Combine all ingredients in a mixing bowl.
2. Form balls using your hands.
3. Place on a baking sheet and cook in a 350°F preheated oven for 10 minutes or until golden brown.

Nutrition information: Calories per serving: 618; Carbohydrates: 6.4g; Protein: 7.1g; Fat: 64.7g; Fiber: 4.2g

Keto Lectin-Free Coffee

Serves: 1
Cooking Time: 3 minutes

Ingredients
- 1 cup organic coffee
- 1 scoop grass-fed butter
- 1 tablespoon coconut oil
- A sprinkle of cinnamon

Instructions
1. On a cup of hot coffee, mix into butter, coconut, oil, and cinnamon.
2. Serve while still hot.

Nutrition information: Calories per serving: 228; Carbohydrates:0 g; Protein: 5.6g; Fat: 38.2g; Fiber: 0g

Indian Samosas

Serves: 8
Cooking Time: 25 minutes

Ingredients
- ¾ cup coconut flour
- ½ teaspoon salt
- 8 ounces grated mozzarella cheese
- 3 tablespoons butter, grass-fed
- 1 onion, chopped
- ¼ teaspoon cumin seeds
- 1 teaspoon garam masala
- ½ teaspoon ground coriander
- 6 ounces cauliflower, chopped
- Salt and pepper to taste
- ¼ cup chopped cilantro

Instructions
1. Create the dough first by combining the coconut flour, salt, and mozzarella cheese.
2. Place in a double boiler and mix with a spatula until all mixture is well-combined.
3. Transfer into a cool counter and knead for 5 minutes. Form balls using your hands and flatten them to form the square samosa wrappers. Set aside.
4. Make the filling. Heat butter in a skillet and sauté the onion, cumin seeds, garam masala and coriander until fragrant. Stir in the cauliflower and season with salt and pepper to taste.
5. Close the lid and simmer for 5 minutes.
6. To assemble the samosa, spoon the filling into the center of the samosa square. Fold it diagonally to form triangles and pinch the edges closed.
7. Place the samosa in a baking sheet and brush with more butter or ghee.
8. Bake in a 350^0F preheated oven for 15 minutes or until golden brown.

Nutrition information: Calories per serving: 96; Carbohydrates: 4.7g; Protein: 4.7g; Fat: 15.1g; Fiber:2.7 g

Stuffed Mushrooms

Serves: 20

Cooking Time: 20 minutes

Ingredients
- 20 large cremini mushrooms, stems removed
- 1 tablespoon melted coconut oil
- 1 cup ground turkey
- 1 head cauliflower, boiled and chopped
- ¼ cup mozzarella cheese
- Salt and pepper to taste
- 4 tablespoons grass-fed butter
- ½ cup chives

Instructions
1. Heat the oven to 400°F.
2. Brush the mushroom caps with coconut oil and place them top-side down on the baking sheet.
3. In a bowl combine the turkey, cauliflower, and mozzarella cheese. Season with salt and pepper to taste.
4. Scoop mixture on the depression in the mushroom cap and brush with butter. Garnish with chives.
5. Bake for 20 minutes.

Nutrition information: Calories per serving: 31; Carbohydrates: 2.4g; Protein: 1.9g; Fat: 10.2g; Fiber: 0.5g

Hard Boiled Eggs

Serves: 6
Cooking Time: 10 minutes

Ingredients
- 6 eggs
- 3 cups water

Instructions
1. Place water and eggs in a pot.
2. Allow to boil for 6 minutes.
3. Turn off the flame and let the eggs remain inside the pot for another 5 minutes.

Nutrition information: Calories per serving: 130; Carbohydrates: 0g; Protein: 4.8g; Fat: 9.6g; Fiber: 0g

Pork Rinds Chicharron

Serves: 6

Cooking Time: 3 hours

Ingredients

- 1 large pork skin, sliced
- 1 ½ teaspoon salt
- 1 teaspoon Chinese five-spice powder
- 3 cups coconut oil

Instructions

1. Season the pork with salt and Chinese five spice powder. Allow to marinate for 2 hours in the fridge.
2. Boil a pot of water and place the pork skin in the boiling water. Cook for 2 hours until the skin is soft. Drain and allow to air dry for a few hours.
3. Heat oil in deep fryer or deep pan over medium flame.
4. Once the oil is hot, fry the pork until crispy.

Nutrition information: Calories per serving:940; Carbohydrates: 0g; Protein: 23.8g; Fat: 109g; Fiber: 0g

Fried Seaweed Snack

Serves: 6
Cooking Time: 2 minutes

Ingredients
- Oil for frying
- 12 nori sheets
- Salt to taste

Instructions
1. Heat the oil in a pan.
2. Once the oil is hot, fry the nori sheets for 1 minute.
3. Allow to drain and season with salt and pepper to taste.

Nutrition information: Calories per serving: 210; Carbohydrates: 1.3g; Protein: 4.6g; Fat: 29.4g; Fiber: 0.2g

Keto Lectin-Free Guacamole

Serves: 6

Cooking Time: 5 minutes

Ingredients
- 4 ripe avocados, pitted and meat scooped
- 1 red onion, minced
- ¼ cup cilantro, chopped
- 1 crushed raw garlic
- ¼ cup freshly squeezed lime juice
- Salt to taste
- ¼ teaspoon cumin

Instructions
1. Combine all ingredients in a bowl.
2. Mash the avocado.
3. Chill in the fridge before serving.

Nutrition information: Calories per serving: 225; Carbohydrates: 14.2g; Protein: 3.0g; Fat: 19.7g; Fiber: 9.4g

Keto Lectin-Free Taco Meat

Serves: 4
Cooking Time: 10 minutes

Ingredients
- 10 teaspoons olive oil
- 1 onion, chopped
- 5 cloves of garlic, minced
- ½ pound ground beef, grass-fed
- Salt and pepper to taste
- 1 teaspoon cumin powder
- 1 teaspoon chipotle powder

Instructions
1. Heat the oil in a skillet and sauté the onion and garlic until fragrant.
2. Stir in the beef and cook for 3 to 5 minutes until golden.
3. Season with salt, pepper, cumin powder, and chipotle powder.
4. Cook for another 5 minutes.
5. Serve with guacamole or on top of lettuce leaves.

Nutrition information: Calories per serving: 225; Carbohydrates: 6.3g; Protein: 7.9 g; Fat: 19.6g; Fiber: 3.2g

Brussels Sprouts Chips

Serves: 3

Cooking Time: 20 minutes

Ingredients
- ½ pounds Brussels sprouts, sliced thinly
- 4 tablespoons olive oil
- 2 tablespoons mozzarella cheese, grated
- 1 teaspoon garlic powder
- Salt and pepper to taste

Instructions
1. Preheat the oven to 400°F.
2. In a bowl, combine all ingredients. Toss to coat the ingredients
3. Place in a baking sheet and bake for 20 minutes or until golden brown.

Nutrition information: Calories per serving:227; Carbohydrates: 5.1g; Protein:15.2 g; Fat: 20.5g; Fiber:3.1 g

Avocado Dip

Serves: 4
Cooking Time: 5 minutes

Ingredients
- 2 ripe avocados, pitted and mashed
- ½ cup coconut milk
- 2 cloves of garlic, minced
- Juice from 1 lime
- Salt and pepper to taste

Instructions
1. Place all ingredients in a mixing bowl.
2. Combine everything and chill before serving.

Nutrition information: Calories per serving: 239; Carbohydrates: 6.7g; Protein: 3.1g; Fat: 21.3g; Fiber: 4.2g

Keto Lectin-Free Fat Balls

Serves: 8

Cooking Time: 5 minutes

Ingredients
- 1 cup shredded coconut
- 1/3 cup ghee
- ½ cup coconut oil
- 2 scoops collagen powder
- 2 tablespoons stevia powder
- 1 teaspoon vanilla extract
- 3 tablespoons water
- ½ teaspoon ground cinnamon
- A dash of salt

Instructions
1. Place all ingredients in a mixing bowl until all ingredients are well-combined.
2. Form small balls with the mixture and place in container.
3. Freeze the balls until ready to consume.

Nutrition information: Calories per serving:192; Carbohydrates: 1.3g; Protein:0.3g; Fat: 21.3g; Fiber: 0.4g

Steak Bites

Serves: 4
Cooking Time: 15 minutes

Ingredients
- ½ cup coconut aminos
- ¼ cup Worcestershire sauce
- 1 teaspoon minced garlic
- 2 tablespoons dried basil
- 1 tablespoon dried parsley
- 1 ½ pounds sirloin steak, cut into 1-inch pieces
- Salt and pepper to taste
- 1/3 cup olive oil

Instructions
1. Place all ingredients in a Ziploc bag and shake to incorporate everything.
2. Marinate for 2 hours in the fridge.
3. Once ready to cook, heat the skillet and pour the steak – marinade and all.
4. Allow to simmer for 10 minutes.
5. Once cooked, allow the sauce to thicken.

Nutrition information: Calories per serving: 504; Carbohydrates: 5.8g; Protein: 15.3g; Fat: 48.2g; Fiber: 2.8g

Made in the USA
Middletown, DE
20 August 2019